I0464557

Look Me In The Eye:

A Complete Guide to Living with Asperger's Syndrome

Introduction

I want to thank you and congratulate you for downloading the book, *"Look Me In The Eye: A Complete Guide To Living With Asperger Syndrome."*

This book contains proven steps and strategies on how to deal with the situation when one of your loved ones is suffering from Asperger Syndrome. Living with Asperger's can be quite stressful and frustrating, especially if you have no idea about the disorder and what to expect when confronted with such a condition.

Asperger Syndrome is not that rare and may afflict any children, regardless of ethnicity, religion, race, and location. Many individuals who have been diagnosed with Asperger's in their childhood have grown up to lead normal lives. However, there are those who never outgrew the symptoms of the disorder. These people lead some degree of normalcy in their lives but have retained the major deficiencies that come with the syndrome: poor communication and social skills. These people probably had not gotten any help from their families and medical professionals — and parents and families play a big role in effectively treating the symptoms of the disorder.

It is important that people with Asperger's receive early diagnosis and intervention, so that they may have a better chance to lead normal lives. Being educated about the syndrome plays a big role, as parents and families of people with Asperger's will better manage the situation after reading this informative book. Valuable information about the syndrome, its various symptoms, causes, prevalence, and treatment will be tackled in this book.

Thanks again for downloading this book, I hope you enjoy it!

Table Of Contents

Chapter 1: Understanding Asperger's Syndrome

Asperger's syndrome is a kind of Pervasive Developmental Disorder (PDD) usually diagnosed during childhood, which is characterized by developmental delay of social skills (to communicate and interact with others), non-verbal communication, lack of empathy, recurring behavioral patterns, and odd preoccupations. Clumsiness, as well as peculiar use of language, has also been noted among people who are diagnosed with the syndrome.

Also known as Asperger's disorder, AS, or Asperger's, Asperger's syndrome was named after Hans Asperger, an Austrian doctor who first defined the condition in 1944. However, it took many years before this particular disorder was recognized for what it truly is.

What is Pervasive Development Disorder?

These are sets of disorders that include impediments in the development of several basic skills, most particularly the capacity to employ the imagination, to interact, and to connect (communicate) with others.

Autism, which has gained popularity due to its established prevalence among children and young adults, is one type of Pervasive Development Disorder. Asperger syndrome is comparable to autism in many different ways. However, there are some notable, vital differences.

How does Asperger's differ from autism?

Although there are various similarities between autism and Asperger's, there are essential differences that characterize the two disorders. For one, children with Asperger's function better cognitively and linguistically than autistic children.

Furthermore, children with Asperger's manifest normal IQs and an almost normal development in language, as odd as their usage of it may sometimes seem.

Causes

At present, the exact cause of Asperger's syndrome has not yet been established. However, there are indications that it is linked to genetics, which means that it is passed on from generation to generation. Nonetheless, this indicator has yet to be proven. Moreover, brain-imaging procedures conducted on people with Asperger's syndrome did not yield any distinct collective pathology.

Treatment

At present, there is no identified single treatment for this type of disorder. The various interventions concocted by experts are meant to improve the symptoms and the functionality of these people in their social circle. Behavioral therapy, however, has been advocated to help people diagnosed with the syndrome overcome their problems in communication and address their clumsiness, as well as their repetitive behavioral patterns. With support and proper treatment, most children with Asperger's eventually improved as they grew older — although difficulties in social interactions and communication may still persist.

The symptoms of this disorder can lead to other severe forms of ailments such as anxiety, depression, obsessive-compulsive disorder, and even aggression, when left untreated. That is why it is imperative that early intervention be given to people diagnosed with the disorder, to avoid complications which can further lead to more severe problems.

Prevalence of Asperger's Syndrome

Asperger's syndrome has just been recently recognized as a particular disorder.

Added to that is the still unclear demarcation whether Asperger's is a variation of High Functioning Autism (HFA) or a distinct disorder. That is why prevalence of this condition cannot be accurately determined. Estimates range from 1 in every 250 to 1 in every 10,000 children in the United States and Canada.

AS is more common than autism though. It has also been reported that males are more affected with the syndrome than females. This disorder can be initially diagnosed among children ages 2 to 6 years old.

As more books and journals have been published about this particular disorder, more diagnostic techniques have also been formulated and carried out, and the estimates of the prevalence of AS have also risen.

Prevention and Cure

There is nothing you can do to ensure that your child will not get Asperger's syndrome. There are no preventive measures to ensure the safety of children from getting afflicted with the disorder. On the other hand, there has also been no identified cure or treatment for the syndrome.

However, there are things that you can do to help your child outgrow the symptoms and live a normal life as an adult, despite some deficiencies in social and communication skills.

Chapter 2: What Are the Symptoms of AS?

Asperger's is characterized not by a particular symptom but by a configuration of symptoms. The indicators of Asperger's syndrome manifest differently from individual to individual and can range from mild to acute. There are various possible symptoms of this disorder but the most vital manifestation is the major difficulty in social settings.

A child with Asperger's syndrome may manifest just a few, several, or all of the indicated symptoms. Hence, no two persons with Asperger's are the same. Indications of the disorder may include the following:

> ➢ **Communication troubles** – A person who suffers from Asperger syndrome may have great difficulty making eye contact when conversing with others. They may also struggle with comprehending language in their usual context since they are usually very literal in their usage of language. They also have trouble interpreting body language and the employment of facial expressions when communicating.

They lack the ability to distinguish slight changes in tone, pitch, and accent which changes the meaning of the other person's speech. As a result, the person may lack the capacity to understand jokes or sarcasm. The speech of one who has AS is also hard to understand since the tone and pitch employed is usually flat and monotonous.

> **Difficulties in social skills** – Children who have Asperger's disorder usually find social interaction difficult. Starting and maintaining conversation is very hard for them. They do not know how to appropriately respond in social situations. Even making friends is not easy for these children. They are also incapacitated by their inability to understand non-verbal cues. They also feel very awkward in social settings.

> **Keen interest on just a few things** – Children with Asperger's Syndrome may develop a very keen interest in a few things such as alarm clocks, video games, computers, televisions, maps, or compasses. This interest can even extend up to the point of obsession.

> **Extreme talents or skills** – Many children who suffer from Asperger's syndrome are extremely talented or skilled in a particular area such as math, arts, or music. They may also exhibit above normal intelligence.

> **Peculiar or recurring behavior** – People with this disorder may cultivate peculiar, repetitive actions like cracking their knuckles, wringing their hands, or twisting their hair. Some children may stand for hours swaying from side to side like a pendulum.

> **Trouble with body coordination** – Children suffering from this disorder may seem gawky and physically awkward most of the times. They are often perceived as generally clumsy due to uncoordinated muscle movement.

> **Unusual fixations or rituals** – Those who suffer from this disorder may nurture habits or practices that they simply refuse to change. These practices may include walking on a particular side of the road or grooming one's self in a particular order. They do not like their routines to be modified or altered. Changing their rituals or routines would be very stressful for them — as well as for you — since they would just resort to some inappropriate behavior.

Chapter 3: How to Diagnose Asperger's Disorder

Don't assume that your child has Asperger's syndrome because he or she has difficulty making friends or interacting with his peers. You must bear in mind that the syndrome is not characterized by any lone symptom but some or all of the identified symptoms. Nonetheless, you should not take the symptom for granted — no matter how insignificant or sporadic it may be.

Asperger's may not be prevented but as a parent or concerned family member, you can do a lot to minimize the ill effects that this particular disorder may result to, if left untreated and undiagnosed. The earlier that Asperger's is diagnosed, the better the chances are to improve the symptoms manifested and retain a semblance of normalcy in the life of an individual with Asperger's syndrome.

Consult a Doctor

However, if your child manifests even some of the identified indicators, you should immediately consult a doctor to ascertain the condition. Expect the doctor to conduct a complete medical history as well as a neurological and physical exam on your child, as part of the evaluation process. Even though there are no particular tests to determine Asperger's, your doctor might employ some tests such as blood tests and X-rays to determine whether there is an underlying physical ailment triggering the symptoms. It is worthwhile to note that many of the children who were diagnosed with AS have been found to have dyspraxia (fine or gross motor coordination disorder) and little muscle tone.

Refer to an Expert

If — after all the examinations and evaluations conducted by your regular doctor are done — no physical ailment is found, the individual may then be referred to a specialist who is trained to detect and cure the syndrome. Such a specialist refers to a medical practitioner who is an expert in childhood development disorders like developmental-behavioral pediatricians, child psychologists or psychiatrists, pediatric neurologists, and other health professionals trained to spot and treat Asperger's syndrome.

The specialist will conduct his or her evaluation based on the level of the individual's development. The specialist's observation of the individual's communication and body language, as well as the capacity to interact with others when placed in a clinical "social setting" study will serve as the basis of his or her diagnosis.

Chapter 4: How Can You Treat Asperger's Syndrome?

At present, a particular cure for Asperger's syndrome has yet to be discovered. However, existing treatments employed by experts may enhance performance and decrease detrimental behaviors. These therapies have been developed to address the fundamental signs of the disorder: compulsive and recurring behaviors, inferior communication abilities, and physical awkwardness.

As mentioned earlier, there is no one particular cure for Asperger's. Nonetheless, experts agree that the earlier the interventions are administered, the better.

Management of the disorder may include a blend of the following treatments:

Psychotherapy of Social Skills

Administered either by a counselor, speech therapist, or psychologist, these remedies are vital means to develop social skills as well as the proficiency to decipher non-verbal hints that is missing in people with Asperger's.

Parent-Family Change of Behavior

This type of treatment actually points to the people surrounding the individual with Asperger's, rather than the individual with Asperger's himself. This means that the people closely associated with the individual who has Asperger's should modify their behavior toward the person in such a way that will strongly encourage positive behavior.

You are not helping your child if you treat him or her with disgust, constant admonitions, verbal abuse, or indifference. Remember that your child has a problem with social skills and communication and not with cognitive abilities. Treating him or her indifferently or negatively will only lead him or her to develop detrimental behaviors which can worsen over time.

Education and Training For The Family and Parents

Considering the pressure and challenge on the families or parents of children with Asperger's, it is crucial that they undergo special training and education to enable them to deal with their AS-diagnosed child better. Reading books that will provide techniques and tips on how to cope with the situation of having a child with Asperger's in the family is also a great help.

As parents or family members of an Asperger's child, you can only extend help to the extent of how informed you are about the condition. You will be in a much better position to provide assistance and help your child live a fairly normal life by learning all about the syndrome.

Specialized Education

Individuals with Asperger's are sent to structured learning sessions meant to provide for their distinctive educational needs. People with this syndrome have special needs that cannot be met in conventional learning systems or settings. This special education is structured in such a way that breaks down tasks into simple, easy-to-follow steps, provides consistent behavior-support, develops the child's interests, and actively captivates the child's attention during organized activities.

Physical and Speech Psychotherapies

These various occupational therapies are structured in such a way that will enhance the functional abilities of children with Asperger's. Depending on the recommendation of your specialist, your child may need to undergo these therapies to help him or her better manage his or her deficiencies.

Medication

There are no specific medications to cure Asperger's disorder as of now. However, there are certain drugs which can be used to treat certain symptoms exhibited by people with Asperger's such as compulsions or preoccupations, depression, aggression, hyperactivity, and anxiety.

For obsessive-compulsive behavior, you can employ the use of tricyclic antidepressants like Clomipramine and various SSRIs (selective serotonin reuptake inhibitors) such as fluoxetine, paroxetine, and fluvoxamine.

For depression, aggression, or irritable behaviors, you can use beta-blockers like propranolol; mood stabilizers such as valproate and lithium; and neuroleptics like olanzapine and haloperidol.

For anxiety attacks, tricyclic antidepressants like imipramine and nortriptylline and SSRIs such as fluoxetine and sertraline are very effective.

For hyperactivity and inattention, pyschostimulants such as destroamphetamine and Strattera like atomoxetine might prove useful.

Chapter 5: Living with Asperger's Syndrome

There is no way you can prevent Asperger's disorder. It can afflict anybody's child regardless of race, ethnicity, social status, location, or religion. However, early detection and intervention of the disorder will give you some leeway in aspiring for a fairly normal childhood and mature life for your child.

Look it in the eye

If your child manifests some of the identified symptoms of Asperger's, deal with it directly. Don't blame yourself or your family's distorted genes for the disorder. Don't blame the child, either. It's not his or her fault for being born that way.

Don't treat or make your child feel as if you think he or she is mentally retarded or deranged, because he or she is not. Children with Asperger's actually have an average to high intelligence quotient. They just lack the ability to effectively communicate and interact with other people.

Accept the condition for what it is but do not disregard it. Your child's normal life in the future depends on how you handle his or her condition. You can choose to either look it in the eye or look away — it's your call. However, if you have come to read this far, it means you are confronting the problem and not pretending that your child does not have AS. There are many things you can do to help alleviate the condition of your child. Accepting that your child has the disorder would be a good start.

Educate your family

You can best help your child by learning all about Asperger's syndrome. Involve everyone in the family in the learning process since they must also deal with the child. Moreover, you need all the help you can get to provide a loving, patient, and supportive environment for your child.

Knowing what to expect and educating yourself about the syndrome is a vital part of helping your child outgrow his symptoms and succeed in things outside of the home.

You can educate yourself and your family by talking to medical professionals who are experts in the treatment and management of Asperger's syndrome, reading literature on AS, and linking up with Asperger's organizations. Through education, you will lessen the stress (not just of your child, but also of you and your family) and be more capable of extending help to your child.

Provide a loving and conducive environment

Children (with disorders or not) will generally thrive when taken care of in a patient, loving, understanding, and supportive environment. This would be an easy task under any normal circumstances. However, dealing with Asperger's syndrome warrants extra patience, determination, and unwavering love and support. It won't be an easy job to live with Asperger's but you can do it if you will yourself to do it.

Your child will have a better chance to have a normal, bright future if you are willing to put up with a little sacrifice: Give him or her more love, patience and understanding. Do not make your child with Asperger's feel out of place in his or her own family. Don't make him or her feel like he or she is living among strangers. Instead, make him feel that he or she really belongs to a family who cares and loves him or her unconditionally, no matter what.

Chapter 6: General Tips and Strategies

It is not easy dealing with a child with Asperger's syndrome, especially if you have no idea about the condition and what to expect in the circumstances. Tempers may flare up, frustrations may set in, and stress may dominate your days if you are not proactive in your role in this particular situation.

Here are some strategies and tips to help you live with Asperger's syndrome:

- Organize a consistent schedule for playtime, homework, meals, bedtime, and other activities. Children with Asperger's syndrome benefit from consistent daily routines and definite rules to follow. When things are done this way, there would be less commotion and stress for the child as well as the family.

- When teaching or imparting lessons to people with Asperger's syndrome, it would be advantageous if you employ the segment-to-whole process method. You see, people with Asperger's have trouble seeing the whole picture and are inclined to see just portions of the whole situation.

- Many individuals with Asperger's don't do well with non-verbal cues; hence, verbal assignments, teachings, and activities would be more appropriate to employ in their case. Handing out instructions in a candid, brief, and direct manner is also beneficial.

- Children with Asperger's may develop an obsessive interest in computers, video games, and other technological devices such as tablets and smartphones. Ensure that they don't have these gadgets in their rooms or else they may end up deprived of regular sleep, which can worsen their symptoms. If they are allowed to use these devices, ensure that their usage is regulated and monitored.

- Try to utilize visual aids as part of conveying instructions and the general learning processes. Using written schedules and other printed materials as part of organizing activities are very valuable tools when dealing with individuals with Asperger's.

- Ensure that there are no background noises during bedtime or study time. Noises like the ticking of the clock, the hum of the air conditioner, or the sound of blinking fluorescent lights will divert the attention of children with AS.

- People with AS have lower tolerance for stressful situations. Try to prepare your child by identifying situations that usually prompt stress and teaching him or her coping skills to better manage the situation.

Transferring to a new home or place, losing someone in the family, or any major change in the family's daily routine are just some of the trigger situations that could generate stress for anyone, but this is especially amplified for a child with Asperger's. Prepare your child for such situations by talking to him or her about such things beforehand and teaching him or her how to deal with it effectively.

- Avoid being harsh on your child. Avoid reprimanding your child with AS to act his or her age. Children with Asperger's syndrome usually mature more slowly than the average child. Learn to be patient with your child's limitations. Focus instead on his or her achievements, no matter how insignificant they may seem to be. Children with Asperger's do have strengths and weaknesses like any other child. Afford him or her all the patience, understanding, support, and love you can muster. The child needs it much more than you'll ever realize.

- It is important that you encourage your child to socialize and interact with people. Teach the child what to do when someone speaks to him or her. Teach him or her the importance of responding to other people when they're trying to talk to him or her. Laud his or her efforts of employing his or her social skills, especially when it's not prompted.

- Teach your child to learn to initiate interaction with other people. Place your child in situations where he or she can practice socializing with others, without being pressured into it.

- Individuals with Asperger's disorder usually lack empathy. You can teach your child to understand other people's feelings through role-playing and discussing the behaviors played afterward. You can also simulate the behaviors and situations you and your child see on television or films. Being open about your feelings will also help your child with AS to emulate you, hence leading him or her to feel empathy for others.

- People with AS will often feel clumsy, awkward, and at a loss when placed in a social situation. Teach your child standard social cues and how to respond appropriately to each of them. Provide him or her with standard responses to standard social cues or you can role-play a scenario to help your child appropriately use his or her communication and social skills when the situation arises.

- Asperger's syndrome is mainly characterized by delays in the development of social and communication skills, as well as muscle coordination in some case. Hence, children with the disorder might not be able to understand social norms that may come naturally to normal children. The child may not understand why people should behave in a certain way. Therefore, it is important that you take time to explain these things and teach him certain rules to enable him to manage his or her social dealings in a much better way.

- Have your child undergo speech or occupational therapy sessions to help with his or her speech or physical impediments. He or she may not understand the employment of these methods so you should explain things before letting him or her attend any session.

- Let your child go to special education classes which are intended to meet his or her special needs. Reinforce his or her learning in the class by monitoring his or her homework and assignments. Assist your child if he or she needs it but let your child do the homework or activity by himself or herself. You are not helping the child if you will do things for him or her.

- Educate your family about everything concerning the syndrome. Teach them what to expect from people with such disorder and how they should appropriately respond to any given situation. You need to extend the education and the change of behavior to all family members since you can't be there all the time. They will have to deal with the family member who has the syndrome, sooner or later. Supporting your child with AS should be a coordinated effort of all family members.

- Lastly, no treatment can be more powerful than a loving, patient, understanding, and supportive family to a child with Asperger's syndrome. Nurture the child with love and understanding. Coupled with the appropriate treatment and interventions, the child with Asperger's will lead a normal adult life in due time.

Conclusion
Do not fill out I will fill out Conclusion myself

Thank you again for downloading this book!

I hope this book was able to help you to understand Asperger's syndrome much more closely.

The next step is to take all the advice in this book and put it to use in your daily life. If you know someone who has Asperger's syndrome, hopefully you now have a better understand of it.

The first step in overcoming any problem is to develop a basic understanding.

Asperger's syndrome is something that should not be taken lightly. It is a very serious issue. You should definitely get outside professional help. They are the ones that can help you the most, but you must be willing to accept it.

There are many different treatment plans to help anybody living with Asperger's. There are resources to help learn social skills. One thing someone can do is just talk to themselves for 5 minutes in front of the mirror to help develop body language and social skills.

There are websites such as RealsocialSkills.com that can teach you about interactions with people and social skills.

You must remember that everything comes with practice and takes time. Nothing worth achieving came overnight. It must be built with hard work and discipline.

There are a lot of agencies that have support and meet ups. You can find some of these resources on Meetup, Craigslist, and Autistic-run organizations in your area, this will provide you with a safe place to make friends and learn social skills.

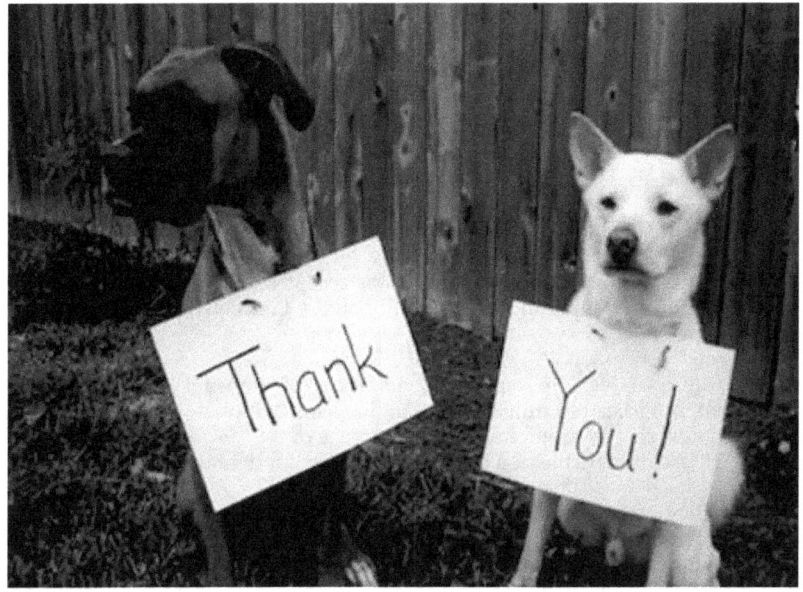

Finally, if you enjoyed this book, then I'd like to ask you for a favor, would you be kind enough to leave a review for this book on Amazon? It'd be greatly appreciated!

Click here to leave a review for this book on Amazon!

Thank you and good luck!

www.ingramcontent.com/pod-product-compliance
Lightning Source LLC
Chambersburg PA
CBHW072253200526
45168CB00015B/1741